Dear Martha,

I want to share Brenner's beautiful thoughts with you. Read them and make them part of you and the coming year can only be fuller & richer.

Love,
Sandy

HEALTH
IS A
QUESTION
OF
BALANCE

HEALTH
IS A
QUESTION
OF
BALANCE

by

Paul Brenner, M.D.

VANTAGE PRESS
New York   Washington   Atlanta   Hollywood

This book is dedicated to all those people who came into
my universe
At the same time that I entered theirs.

FIRST EDITION

Copyright © 1978 by Paul Brenner, M.D.

Published by Vantage Press, Inc.
516 West 34th Street, New York, New York 10001

Manufactured in the United States of America
Standard Book Number 533-03513-9

Contents

INTRODUCTORY

Everything is the same;
There is nothing original.
So if perchance I used your aphorism,
Thank you for bringing it to my consciousness.
It will appear in this book with both our love.

There is order and meaning to each of our lives.

Autobiographical Milestones of My Work

1) Born
2) Buddy's death
3) Decision to become a doctor
4) Twenty more years of school
5) Father's death
6) Obstetrics and gynecology
7) Cancer fellowship
8) Andy's death
9) The Women's Movement
10) Free clinics
11) Acupuncture
12) Russ's death
13) The Moody Blues
14) Meditation
15) Isolation Tank Experience—John Lilly
16) Fasting
17) Meadowlark—Evarts Loomis
18) Guatemala earthquake
19) Decision to leave traditional medicine
20) Intensive Journal Work—Ira Progoff
21) Brugh Joy
22) Elisabeth Kubler-Ross
23) My family: Joyce, Brad, Elisabeth, Ilene, Anne, Sybil, Claire
24) All

People are seeking a total physician.

I am seeking a total patient.

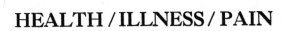

HEALTH / ILLNESS / PAIN

Health is no more than a question of balance.

Health is the balance between hypo- and hyper- states of illness. It is that range of normalcy between two comparatively polarized states.

For example:

Hypothyroid—normal thyroid—Hyperthyroid
Hypotension—normal blood pressure—Hypertension
Hypoglycemia—normal sugar metabolism—Diabetes
etc.,

Dishealth occurs in that millisecond that an individual puts himself/herself down for being anything less than perfect—

And therefore,
health and dishealth are in a constant state of flux.

Imbalance in favor of dishealth occurs when the mind refuses to relinquish self-deprecating thoughts.

Stress can shift the fulcrum of balance from health
to dishealth—if readjustment is delayed
then disease serves as the new center of stability.

Therefore,
stress is anything that alters the course of human events. If understood, it can serve as a prime mover in seeking out one's destiny and if not appreciated, as the initiator of dishealth. In a sense it is responsible for man's impermanence.
It is not unlike the wind that drives the sailboat—we need it to reach our destination, but when the gale force pervades then one should take down the sail, acknowledge the wind and let it pass. . . .

Stress sets the stage for illness—
There are viruses and bacteria on the page you're reading—
If zapped—

Don't shout *Why Me!!*
But ask why me?
in silence

Suffering has the propensity to heighten one's awareness—

Do you need a heart attack or—cancer
to make today count?

There is the external manifestation of disease—
but to treat, one must learn the internal chronology.
What is happening in your life to allow illness?

Stress does not have to be negative in context—
even celebrating Christmas can disrupt the balance.

Unresolved stress sets the stage for illness.

Illness is a friend.

If one accepts illness and finds meaning in it and establishes obtainable goals, then the illness ceases to be illness and now is transmuted to health.

Health does not mean freedom from disease—it means understanding and acceptance of the life process.

Illness has the potential to place one in a higher state of consciousness. It may provide the opportunity to exercise options and establish priorities—

It's an internal psychiatrist—use it—you paid for it.

Acute illness is cause and effect—

If one has a clear vision as to the cause,
then it is easily treatable.

Chronic illness is an effect whose cause has
been modified by time—

If treatment precedes understanding of the cause
then the cure may be only temporary
or
one illness will beget another illness.

The malingerer is fixated in a childhood where more strokes were given for illness and pain than for simply
being.

What are you getting out of illness that you can't achieve in health?

Illness is blocked love.

Isometric exercises increase blood pressure by producing a sustained block in blood flow.

Illness is a sustained block to the universal flow of love.

Therefore, illness can be caused by non-acceptance or non-relinquishment of love.

Misinterpretation of love is the bottom line in the causality of illness.

Perception, interpretation and recall of pain are man's most primitive survival mechanisms—

if overplayed they can become the disease itself and be retained as memory.

Pain and disease are static on a tape. To deal with it one must interpret the tape long enough to allow the previous normal memory of health to be heard.

At the moment of regained health man becomes ethereal— he returns to the pure state for which he was intended.

Get in touch with that feeling of well-being and use it as a mantra.

For some, pain is an affirmation of life.

("Pinch me so I know I am not dreaming")

For others, pain and disease are not only the chief complaints but a cause. It is a possession that cannot be shared. It may become so contracted and introspective that with time and repetition, it serves as a negative mantra to achieve meditative despair.

Variety in behavioral patterns can change
the outcome of a negative tape.

THANK YOU, ALBERT EINSTEIN

Try concentrating on the person in the car in front of you
and you will be amazed how often he will turn around,
maybe because
 Thought is mass
  and therefore
Unshared thoughts are possessions.

Unexpressed thoughts are no different from mass—
they are congealed energy.

In thinking of others—*please*
only have thoughts of love.

Power is non-sharing.

There is no difference between thoughts
and bombs.

From health to illness is not progressive—
it is a quantum leap—
it is a discontinuous relationship.

As light cannot be accounted for by oscillations of atoms which take place in a continuous manner, one cannot account for the oscillation of the mind/body between disease and health as a progressive or continuous one.

It is discontinuous depending on a definite quantum of energy to produce one or the other state.

If this proposition is accepted and imbalance of
body or mind is dishealth,
then the upper or lower limit of normal range for
health should be treated with exercise, diet and
meditation, for a minimal increment beyond this range
produces disease—
and if likened to the quantum theory, then the amount
of energy or therapy needed to reverse the process is
a multiple of the minimal increment that produced it.

Acute illness is cause and effect and can be viewed
as a straight line between the two events of
health and illness.
Chronic illness is disease spread over a
period of time and is subjected to space-curvature.
It is Riemann's Geometry.

The space-curvature is created by man viewing his
expectations over time.

Expectations are the subatomic particles of belief systems.

The degree to which man holds on to his expectations is directly proportional to the force of his gravity.

To transcend either a belief or expectation only leads to a new set of "what is."

Therefore the only way to fly is to be in a constant state of letting go—

For a physician or patient to observe chronic illness in a Newtonian cause and effect manner is preposterous.

Simultaneity may be approximate in acute illness, but misses its mark in chronic illness.

It is not only the self-imposed expectation that affects disease, but the expectations of other bodies that surround that individual's universe.

It is in this situation that non-causal factors affect causality— *i.e.,* Jungian synchronicity.

Although it may appear obvious, I feel it is worth stating that recovery is a function of the interval between onset of disease and its appropriate therapy—*i.e.,* don't waste time—get to it.

Social and personal stresses are not unlike the subatomic particles in Brownian movement. They are not in the spectrum of our visibility but have the propensity to alter our path and assure our impermanence. The agitation is not good or bad—it is relative.

If we can accept the Field Theory of Matter then there is no such thing as "My space." Space is co-habited.

"I need my own space" is not only materialistic; it is impossible.

Mass is no more than congealed energy, so the more chronic the illness, the more energy is consumed—the more the mass.

Depression or disease may be no more than not enough energy to move mass.

Forgive me, Albert.

But if $e = mc^2$ where energy = mass times the constant of the velocity of light squared, and since the above formula is symbolic of a relative relationship,

then can one extrapolate from these symbols: $e = B \times M^2$ where energy = the mass of body times the velocity of the mind squared (right x left hemisphere)?

Then is it possible that the mind of the catatonic or comatose person is moving at such high velocity that the mass of the body is not only increased but there is not enough energy to overcome the inertia of the mass? Perhaps they are stuck in another form of reality different from ours. The treatment is mutual unsticking through acceptance of other reality systems. Is it possible that death occurs at that instant when the velocity of the mind approaches the speed of light?

Is that why in the various stages and types of anaesthesia and meditation as the mind becomes free, the body assumes a feeling of heaviness?

I really don't know!—Do you?

Death occurs when there is not enough energy to continue
or reverse the life process—
But

since energy cannot be created or destroyed, then
death returns matter back to a free state—

Unity.

If frequency can affect quanta and frequency is the number of repetitive events over a given period of time—then frequency is analogous to memory.

The mind is a totality of our experiences—

It is the distance traveled in relationship to the time that it has taken us to get there which in turn is a function of our velocity of understanding.

Therefore, age is not necessarily wisdom.

Isn't it interesting that Einstein's theory of relativity was based on the understanding of light transmission?

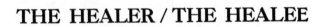

THE HEALER / THE HEALEE

Doctor-patient therapy should be based on a broad situational ethic. That is to say, the need of the situation should dictate the specific therapy to meet the particular needs of the individual. This would embrace not only the traditional forms of western medicine, but would integrate them with alternative therapies in a complementary manner.

The new medicine is called holistic medicine, but the clinic for holistic treatment is the clinic Earth. It's all out there already. There is no need to institutionalize it.

The future of medicine is a place where technology and the metaphysical (that which hasn't been explained by technology) can co-exist—where an individual can find either traditional medicine or the esoteric or both, depending on that individual's transcendent beliefs.

The holistic center, if designed, should be a gigantic magnifying glass that shows each individual not only alternatives, but their place in society and their symbiotic relationship with the earth. The center should be a place where the word "best" doesn't exist. It is not found in the rhetoric of the evolved. If the clinic is designed to deal with an infinite number of probabilities of belief, then it becomes free from comparison.

Science in its structure is a double-edged sword.
At the moment it tells you what can be accomplished,
it also states what cannot be effected.

The mystical is abstract and there provides hope.

Should physicians deny hope?

Integration of the spiritual and scientific is an
obtainable reality.
There is no conflict!

Many people want to "beat" the problem
themselves—but competition always produces at least
one loser—
sometimes all of us need a little assistance.

If your therapy isn't working, see a physician. If it's not
working with traditional medicine, do whatever feels
good. Feeling good is the first twist in changing the
combination to your locked-in memory.

Remember, the memory of previous health is there.

Listen in silence.

Three Types of Response to Cancer

Denial   —"Impossible—it's a mistake—I don't have it." This response has minimal effect on the disease course.

Attack   —"I'll beat it" which has mild to moderate effect on longevity.

Acceptance—"I know what I have, but I must get out of the hospital to finish my work" which may have profound effect on longevity.

Setting obtainable goals is paramount to quality of survival.

The external healer opens a set of belief systems which were previously impervious to recovery.

The external healer is the guide who allows the internal healer (patient) to transcend the belief system of what *is*.

The healer and the healee are the same person.

The primary gate in healing is the gate of acceptability,
that is, do you accept the premise
that the healer is offering you?

If you do, then you are involved in both processes.
If your gate doesn't swing both ways, get a carpenter.

If psychosomatic illness is an accepted disease entity, then why can't we learn psychosomatic recovery from disease and practice psychosomatic health daily?

When a type of therapy does not appear to be successful—
you can only say that it did not work at that time with
that therapist—

It does not negate its potential value for you or for
someone else in the future.

Traditional medicine / acupunture / polarity / *shiatsu* / massage / faith healing / etc.
all have a common denominator in their success—

1) total concentration on the moment
2) determination of the cause
3) internalization of the imagery of what is happening
4) acceptance of what was offered
5) appreciation of what was done

If acupuncture works on animals—
what makes us so special?

Is there a possibility that lower animals are more
accepting—if yes, are they lower?

If a man can be identified by his fingerprint,
Then why can't one be diagnosed by looking at one's iris?
Or healed by placing a needle in the ear
Or by massaging the foot—

Is not the egg the entire chicken?

The physician's desk reference should include acupuncture, meditation, imagery, psychotherapy, yoga, *tai chi,* diet, exercise programs, etc.—
rather than just a host of medications based on effect with minimal relationship to cause.

Tips to the Patient

Remember you're the one who gives permission to be helped or exploited.

Help the doctor and yourself by accepting your own responsibility for health.

Life is an appreciation—

All is for naught in unthinking methodology.

If you run to relieve anxiety, then you're taking your anxiety out on your body. You may save yourself a trip to the cardiologist but end up in the orthopedist's office.

Running should be for the sole purpose of the love and appreciation of running.

If you can't get out of bed to exercise—

Stretch like a cat

Imagine yourself doing simple exercises with your eyes closed.

Use those limbs that move.

Love those that don't.

Imagery works!

Tips to Doctors

Educate the patients to a level at which they can select appropriate therapy based on their belief.

To raise the patient's consciousness is to lower one's malpractice.

If a placebo works 35% of the time, why not use more nothing.

An X ray that is shown to a patient can be used two ways—

1) diagnosis
2) a biofeedback mechanism through imagery to enable that individual to visualize recovery.

If it is used only to validate the cause, it may serve only to reinforce a negative process.

Statistics are valid for Wall Street—

But for that person who recovers or dies it's 100%.

Statistical proof is an outgrowth of materialism. One must see it and own it before one can believe it.

We can't accept love because we can't own it; how can we rely on just feelings?

Worse still, what if we don't get back our investment?

How can we prove a humanistic approach to medicine will effect therapy?

The physician must walk the tight-rope between being an observer and a participant.

If only the former, one may miss the mark, while if only the latter one may become the mark.

If the duality of observer—participant is achieved, then the key to health—*COMPASSION*—is reached.

Self-Healing

Doing and perceiving are in conflict.
(Ever try to tickle yourself? It doesn't work.)

So set your intention.
Then, let it go.

Do-It-Yourself Psychiatry

If life is a mirror of your mind—then talk to it.

    Talk to your
    work
    body
    society
    loved ones
    hates
    Talk, talk, talk

But if you talk / you must listen

                    Listen to your
                    work
                    body
                    society
                    life
                    loved ones
                    hates
                    Listen, listen, listen

Remember
in the preceding two pages
it's a dialogue between two monologues, each with
its own identity—discussed in silence.

Meditation is talking to oneself in a monologue.

In silence one can hear

Creativity is applied intuition—

It is no more than doing what one is intended to do.
It is the unfolding and the fulfillment of the self.

In the end, who is responsible for health?

Maybe the mirror will explain!

Responsibility means personal involvement in the present—not blame for the past.

PHILOSOPHY

PEOPLE ARE BORN AND PEOPLE DIE
  AND IN THE STILL POINT OF THAT
  EXISTENCE IS BEING.
AS A TREE—
  THE LIMB NO LONGER RECOGNIZES
  THE TRUNK.
THERE IS A DISSOCIATION
  THERE IS HEALTH WHICH IS ETHEREAL.
NO HANDS / LEGS / EYES
  IT IS WHAT IS NOT.
THERE IS ILLNESS
  PALPABLE / PERCEIVABLE
  IT IS WHAT IS.
THE BALANCE IS THE STILLPOINT OF WHAT IS
AND WHAT IS NOT
  WHAT IS—IS WHAT IS NOT
WHAT IS NOT—IS WHAT IS
  A UNIT OF ONE.
HEALTH SEEKS UNITY BY BEING WHAT IS
  DISEASE SEEKS UNITY BY BEING WHAT IS
  NOT
WHEN ONE SEPARATES THE ONE
  THERE IS NONE
IN THE END—TO BE RESPONSIBLE FOR ONESELF
  ONE MUST APPRECIATE
WHAT IS NOT APPRECIATED.

We are all ethereal beings—
Why do we need pain to make us feel human?

As you are reading, you probably are unaware of your
    thumb—
Is it necessary to put it in the door to appreciate it?

Ode To Thumbs

Since opposition of the thumb separates primates
from other animals
                    and
since the thumb has the greatest relative representation
of all body parts in the motor/sensory area of the brain
                    and
since the fetal hands appear to move more freely in the
pregnant uterus than any other bodily part
                    then perhaps
it could explain why those areas of the perfectly flexed fetal
body that are most easily touched by the hand have
proportionately greater representation in the brain
than areas that cannot be reached.
                    Then maybe that's why
hand and thumb position are so important in prayer and
meditation
                    and maybe that's why
the major therapeutic site for acupuncture is the thumb.
                    If so
stroking your thumb when you have head and neck
     problems may give you some relief by overloading the
     brain input.
                    If so
then thumb sucking may not be for oral gratification
but for thumb gratification
                    If so
                    Thumbs up!
Appreciate the healing power of your hands.

To understand one thing is to understand all things.

Roy Lichtenstein utilizes many dots of equal size to form figurative art—not unlike looking at a comic strip under a magnifying glass.

Each dot is a universe within itself, but the dot cannot exist isolated from the picture or the figure without the dot. As with men, all the dots appear the same—they are equal.

Each dot, as man, also has its own space. Yet there is a limitation to how far a dot can move before it distorts the picture—there is balance.

Uniqueness lies not in the events of one's life as much as in the path between events.

People are like a jar of chocolate-covered raisins—

They may each appear to be on different levels, but each tastes as sweet.

Life is like pinball—

You come out of darkness as a sphere.

Although knocked around, you try to
light up as many lights as possible
along your unique path.

As in all contests you're playing
against yourself.

You only lose if you tilt (go out of
balance) —and then must pay
to play again.

You reenter darkness to play another
game at another time and follow a path
in another space.

Utopia:

A place where stress factors are constantly being monitored and a resocialization process begins when the body "tilts."

Utopia:

A place where a person can be educated to the level of the teacher in order to accept responsibility for decision-making—and then becomes the teacher.

Utopia:

A place where the credit for healing resides with the healed.

Utopia:

A place where man will accept all the notes without comparing one octave to another,

    and finally,
A place where self-love will not be considered egotistical.

One loves all things in loving oneself!

The mind and body are similar to a computer—each is only as good as the information you put in.

Unlike the computer, the mind does not have to be programmed by an outside source, but at times it sure may help.

If we assume that our mind computer is imprinting every millisecond, then the computer has three alternatives:

intended storage
non-intended storage
no storage.

Consciousness is intended storage while awareness is the sum total of intended storage and non-intended storage.

If you're lucky you have no storage, then each moment becomes a new creative process.

Western medicine makes the mistake of treating what comes into consciousness and not what comes into awareness.

Biofeedback is the conversion of unconscious programs to a conscious level and replay for intended storage.

Where do yogis hide their machine?

Polarization creates a diadic God.

Polarization is the death of wisdom.

Without bad, one cannot appreciate good; therefore, bad is good!

In all things one can find a combination of opposites—
Women tend to be internally liberated and externally
inhibited, while men
tend to be externally liberated and internally inhibited.

Both need to be liberated, but in seeking the balance
between internal and external freedoms, beware that the
gain on one side is not reflected by the loss on the other.

Interpretation of a symbol is its negation.

How you feel about a symbol is its essence.

There is no difference between the awake and dream state.

The objects that one witnesses with eyes open or closed are no more than guideposts to inner vision / wisdom.

If one can buy this premise, then the blind man may see as much in life or perhaps more than the person with 20/20 vision.

Fads are crystals of awareness that have overshot their mark.

I pray that the awareness groups of the seventies will not become the religious wars of the nineties.

If you have it—keep it.

If you have to justify it—
you lose it.

There are many different paths which share the same identical subatomic particles and therefore are reflections of all paths.

To be a winner—one must be willing to lose.

In that moment of decision to take the option, you win either way. For you have one less thing to think about. . . .

Ants constantly bump into each other and in so doing transfer knowledge, which is called trophallaxis (the social enzyme).

Man can learn from all creatures big or small.
But first he must learn to touch.

We guard our knowledge to give ourselves worth.
In so doing we prevent space for anything else
and lose freedom.

Knowledge without understanding is not unlike
an "over-the-counter" decongestant—
temporary relief.

The word "if" gives you permission to do what you always wanted to do—

> If I were thinner, I'd have . . .
> If my back were better, I'd have . . .
> *ad nauseam!*

The only way to legitimize our plight is to create our own fears.

Hate serves the purpose of allowing one to focus on something other than oneself, while love serves no one's purpose.

Alchemy

The resolution of the monad is the diad—
The resolution of the diad is the triad—
The resolution of the triad is the monad—

And so to the next level of awareness. . . .

THERE IS THE TRINITY IN ALL THINGS.

The trinity is the point between opposites that produces balance, strength and unity.

The third element is no more than the alchemy of the other two.

It may be a line drawn from the apex of an equilateral triangle through its base forming right angles—the cross—

or

the balance between two opposing equilateral triangles—the star of David—

or

the strength produced by the curvature that unites the two radii of a circle.

It is the point between man and God—

It is man in God and God in man.

The essence of the Trinity/equilateral triangle is infinite. . . .

BALANCE / LOVE / DEATH / ENLIGHTENMENT

Man's past, when analyzed, points to the future
but is only viewed in balance by being
in the present.

The degree one focuses backward or forward
is the degree that one suffers.

How many people
can see themselves in a Polaroid picture
60 seconds after it was taken and say,
"That's how I used to look."

When someone compliments you—accept it.
Don't block your birthright with indignant modesty.

You are where you are because of where you have been—
so don't knock it.

Life is a bowl of cherries—only for that moment / for those
cherries / in that bowl.

The western ethic that a man's reach should exceed his grasp deters man from dealing effectively with those obtainable phenomena within his immediate reach.

Man's task is to "de-evolve" and return to newborn bliss—accepting all things and radiating love.

When giving and receiving are achieved simultaneously healing and rebirth occur.

The Tao is the path in life that makes you feel warm—
at love with all things—
part of all things—
it is heart level.

Man's will is a double-edged sword that allows him to direct his destiny on the one hand; in that same moment of self-determination there is an equal loss of oneness with the universe.

His task is to achieve the duality of movement and non-movement—what the Taoist refers to as the STILL POINT.

There is meaning and order in all things—
stop and smell the roses.

One fears death tomorrow if one hasn't lived life today.

Man is motivated to accomplish through fear of death.

Striving for possessions is no more than a way of holding on.
. . . Hoping that all that junk will prevent you from falling
through the hole.

There is more to life than living.

Life is just a parable unless
it has been experienced.

The only ones who suffer in death are the living.

To love is to open.

To get the message, one has only to open the envelope—
then share the knowledge.

For only in unconditional sharing, can the giving and
receiving fuse into one.

Love is to open oneself
to all things without
holding on to anything—

It is synonymous with meditation.

It is synonymous with healing.

In the silence of meditation

You may hear birds, people, cars
Have thoughts of rocks, trees
Sensation of a breeze
The smell of a rose
The recall of an argument or a hate

But through meditation you are
The birds, the people, the cars, the rocks
The breeze, the rose
The recall of an argument, the hate
With the realization that you are all of the above
You can now open your eyes and
See for the first time.

Now you are the meditation.

Why do we show more love to our fellowman
in sickness than in health?

Enlightenment is love.

It is seeing perfection in all things.

The first ray of love must be for oneself. This is followed by the clarity of insight that reveals that if I am perfect then all that surrounds me is perfect.

Even our "screw-up" cannot be a more perfect "screw-up"; accept it as such.

Man's task is to learn from those self-imposed pratfalls.

Upon confrontation with a given obstacle, the observer must view the event as a learning experience that time will wash away.

Enlightenment is freedom from comparison—
    There is no black / no white / no shade—
    It is pure light undisturbed by prisms—
    Undefined by wavelengths.
Without comparison there is unity.

How do you know when you're illumed?

When you're fused with the moment.

Am I enlightened?

Only if you are!

You and I are the way—

We are part of all movements.

The guru you're searching for is you.

Please fill in the following pages—as the starting point for your own book. Then after experiencing each page, you're ready to share it with a friend and in so doing free yourself for new thoughts.

And a new book.